MEDICARE WARS:
A Radical New Approach
Learn
Fight
Win

By
Charlene Brash Sorensen
Peggy Bechko

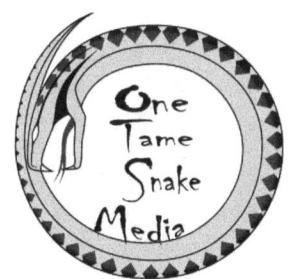

The information in this pamphlet was accurate to the best of the Authors knowledge upon its initial publication date.

TABLE OF CONTENTS

Dedication

This pamphlet is dedicated to Thomas Paine (1737-1809)—a Revolutionary War hero who was a journalist, writer, and political philosopher. During 1775-1776, Paine wrote and then published a 48-page pamphlet entitled "Common Sense". He wanted the settlers of America to think about what was happening and to fight for independence against the unfair and the unjust British King and Parliament.

The Authors of *this* pamphlet (with more to come) believe he had the "right" of it in urging American's to "think about" what was happening.

"The cause of America is in a great measure the cause of all mankind. Many circumstances have, and will arise, which are not local, but universal, and through which the principles of all Lovers of Mankind are affected, and in the Event of which, their Affections are interested."

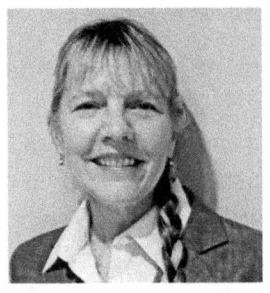

Charlie Brash-Sorensen

I **_NEVER_** imagined being compelled by a sense of justice, compassion for others, and outrage to pick up once more the mantle of "Medicare expert". But on November 9, 2016 my past work caught up with me 1,455 miles from where I left it on the Olympic Peninsula outside Seattle, Washington. The following morning the regressive Republican Party openly declared war on Medicare—our Medicare.

How did I get here?

I have relocated across country since my last employment "gig" in 2012. I took up a children's book writing project with my one of my best friends. I got an Irish setter puppy that has become a big dog. I bought a house after renting for 8 years. My husband retired and then returned to work full-time. I was asked to join a book club. I paid for a gym membership that I actually use. In March 2017 I turn 65 years old and will be eligible for Medicare.

What makes me an "expert"?

Twenty-six years in management and executive positions in the Medicare and Medicaid health insurance industry is a LONG time. It takes a toll personally, emotionally and physically. It takes a few years to totally drop the stress and move on. In my particular case shedding my career persona:

- Director of Strategic Planning
- Director of Operations
- Associate Executive Director
- Vice President of Network Development
- Vice President of Operations
- Chief Compliance Officer
- Senior Consultant in a highly respected nation consulting firm

—has taken 4 years.

To be completely honest, I continued to participate in professional organizations, attended a few seminars, and read endless Medicare pamphlets - some little voice inside kept telling me to "stay in touch". Now I know why.

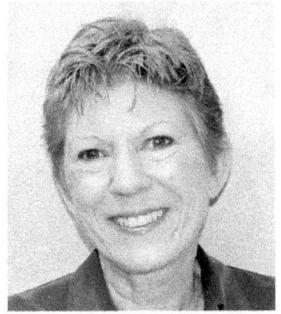

Peggy Bechko

As we get older, probably for the first time our attention turns to things like Medicare and retirement. It would be better if we paid attention when you're younger, but well, there you are.

All of this means an incredible learning curve just about the time you think you're about done with all that and can relax a bit. I mean there's so much else you want to learn about so who has room to cram all this junk into our brains?

The relaxing part was true for my grandparents, but not for us. Things were pretty straight-forward for them, but politics over the decades has created a monster called Medicare with all its parts and subparts. It truly is enough to make you want to throw your hands up and give up. But wait, I can't do that, and neither can you. We have to take care of ourselves despite the apparent desire of our own government to do us in.

I mean look, these two guys want to partner up and destroy this already confusing plan we've all paid into most or all of our lives; Medicare —

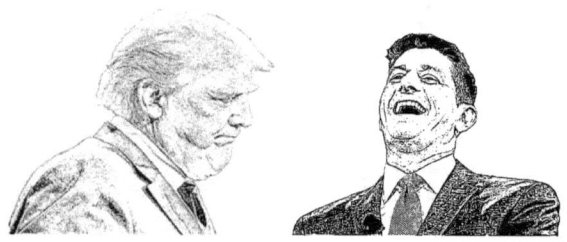

Luckily for me, I have a great friend, co-author of this, and the pamphlets on Medicare to follow. She worked in the insurance industry for years and knows the ins and outs and frightening turns health care can take at this time of life courtesy of the country we live in where we have a 'for profit' health care system.

So I went to her and I said, "Charlene, what the F*&!#%!!!! Help!"

And she did.

So now it's our combined goal to help you with short books in bite-size pieces that will clear things up for you. Or at least filter out a bit of the silt.

Now I've been a professional writer for most of my life (fiction, non-fiction articles and screen scripts).

Meanwhile Charlene has spent most of her career working with these ridiculous HMO plans.

Between us we decided it would be a great idea to break this whole mess down into those bite-sized pieces that 'regular' people might actually understand. Or, if not that, then at least help steer people in the right direction that will benefit them the most while confronting this beast. Suggestions, links, warnings; everything we can think of to help the Medicare recipient.

Introduction

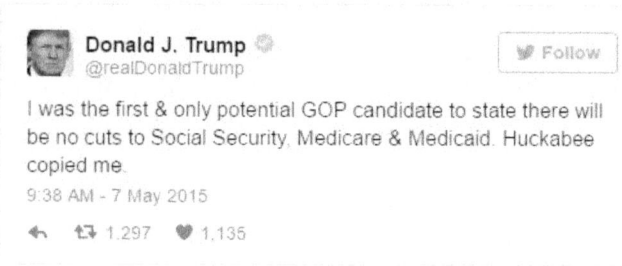

The Authors believe the above campaign promise is one Donald Trump (Trump) does not intend to keep. It is our task as citizens to hold Trump to his word. Shredding the current Medicare health care system and selling it to the highest bidder does not "promote the general welfare" as guaranteed in the Preamble to the "Constitution".

Who Should Read These Pamphlets

1. THOSE who are willing to take action to save Medicare from private insurance companies;
2. THOSE who want to learn and understand how Medicare currently works;
3. THOSE who believe that a "Medicare For All" program is a potentially viable universal health insurance option for every American.

What We Face

Simply put, present and future Medicare beneficiaries face a hostile and regressive Republican Congress bent on changing the current program to further financially benefit private insurance companies, large multi-national pharmaceutical firms, and hospital corporations. Scrapping the current Medicare program and placing it in the hands of "big business" is simply put—Wrong.

Let us be very clear. Members of Congress, whose goal is to privatize Medicare, have no interest in your health care except as it may financially benefit themselves and their corporate stakeholders (a person or business that has invested money in something. The latter group includes: insurance **firms**, pharmaceutical **companies**, and hospital **corporations**. In a for-profit world your health and well-being is simply a bottom-line number on a corporate profit-and-loss statement.

The average American will always come out last in a government controlled (or influenced) by firms, companies and corporations that have the goal of creating laws that benefit their bottom-line.

Finally, those politicians intent on handing over Medicare to "private" companies are purposefully using language to confuse and influence the uneducated and the under-educated. You will hear politicians, journalists, "talking heads", and "think tanks" say about Medicare bankruptcy - which is not true unless your politician makes it happen!

These stakeholders will publish articles with deceptive headlines meant to persuade the average recipient Medicare insolvency is imminent unless drastic changes are made. Article titles and content will use misleading words such as "empowering", "premium support", and "modernization" to calm concerns. Titles will scream frightening language such as "Medicare Bankruptcy Looms".

The Truth Hurts

Health care is an "industry". To grow, industries require profits. Health care is "for profit" though it may cloak itself in the title of "not-for-profit". Health care business stakeholders speak about people on Medicare as consumers—users of products that just so happen to be products related to health care. Health care "providers" sell their products to the consumer in exchange for money.

Those CEO's and corporate board members of companies that will profit from a "private" Medicare program will *never* be in a position where they face personal bankruptcy and long-term poverty due to impossible to pay premiums, deductibles, co-insurance, and copayments required for necessary medical and pharmaceutical care. That firm's CEO will *never* have to stand in your shoes. That industries corporate board member will *never* understand the choices you may have to make between eating and paying for chemotherapy.

Their wealth and privilege protect them from these choices. Their wealth and privilege permit them to view your dilemma in a cold-hearted and disinterested manner.

For *some perspective*...here are the 2015 CEO salaries of the 5 largest health insurers:

Company	Salary + Other Compensation
CIGNA	$17.3 million
Aetna	$17.3 million
UnitedHealth Group (United Healthcare)	$14.5 million
Anthem	$13.6 million
Humana	$10.3 million

And for just a *bit more perspective*, two hospital "non-profit" CEO's earned nearly $10 million dollars in 2014:

Michael Dowling of Northwell Health (Great Neck, New York) earned $9.6 million while George Halvorson of the Kaiser Foundation earned $9.8 million. And please do not give me that tired and unfounded old argument that a not-for-profit hospital or insurance company needs to pay a lot of money in order to attract talent—that just has not been proved to be true. These are some pretty big pay days for not-for-profit hospitals that **don't pay taxes.**

And while we are at it some *final perspective*, how about those BigPharma CEO salaries:

Company	CEO Salary + Other Compensation
Bristol-Myers Squibb	$26.1 million
Merck (recently merged with Schering-Plough)	$21.4 million
Johnson & Johnson	$20.4 million
Pfizer (recently merged with Wyeth)	$18 million
Abb Vie*	$17 million

*A 2013 spin-off from Abbott Labs.

Here is a brief list of drugs manufactured and sold by these pharmaceutical companies and frequently prescribed for Medicare recipients:

Liptor – cholesterol
Lyrica – nerve pain

Celebrex – arthritis
Viagra
Enbrel – anti-inflammatory
Singulair – asthma
Cozaar – high blood pressure
Remicade – arthritis
Humira – anti-inflammatory
Coumadin – prevent blood clots
Pravachol - cholesterol

Medicare has flaws. In the opinion of the Authors, these flaws need to be addressed, fixed or changed but not by selling Medicare to the highest bidder. Right now, Medicare works just fine for 55,504,005 enrollees (2015, Kaiser Family Foundation).

So…let's keep it that way for now and in the experienced hands of Social Security, the Department of Health and Human Services (DHHS), and the Centers for Medicare and Medicaid Services (CMS).

If You Choose To Do Nothing

1. Medicare covered health and pharmacy benefits will decrease;
2. Medicare premiums, deductibles, co-insurance and copayments (medical and pharmaceutical) will increase to unaffordable levels once current regulatory controls are lifted;
3. Medicare out-of-pocket expenses for

catastrophic care may well push beneficiaries into financial disaster;

4. Congress, the media, and corporate stakeholders will portray Medicare beneficiaries as selfish and greedy—taking money from the hardworking taxpayer due to their sense of "entitlement.

4. Congress will promote the idea that Medicare costs are jeopardizing their ability to have a "balanced budget" without "increasing taxes".

If You Choose To Do Something

If you get educated and if you get involved, the War on Medicare can be won.

Pamphlet Goals

<u>Format</u>

The Authors selected the "pamphlet" format for three reasons:

1. Pamphlets are generally short and to the point;
2. Pamphlets provide bite-sized information making ideas easier to understand;
3. Pamphlets are relatively quick to produce.

This format allows us to rapidly provide our readers with the knowledge and tools to act in opposition to changes to drastically alter Medicare and to sell it on the private market.

<u>Two Goals</u>

Almost everyone has heard of Medicare. Well...maybe not a twenty-something...but "most". We also hope to reach Readers who haven't given Medicare a thought because it so far in the future. The Authors believe that, not only should Medicare be preserved as a government-controlled program for current users, but that it is a viable "universal" health care option for all Americans.

Six *Medicare Wars* pamphlets are planned. Our goals are modest:

1. **Education**. Every reader needs to know how the current Medicare program works. Readers also need a few pieces of data to help them understand the program – how it's paid for, the number of people receiving benefits, etc.

2. **Call To Action (CTA)**. It does no good to learn how Medicare works today unless the reader is willing to DO SOMETHING (or several somethings) to hold onto the program—and possibly extend it to all Americans.

Frankly, if you have downloaded or purchased this first pamphlet and are not interested in both goals—You do not belong here.

Before We Begin

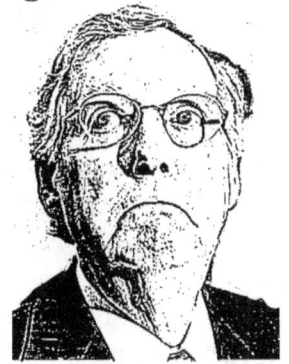

Mitch McConnell
(Republican)
Speaker of the Senate

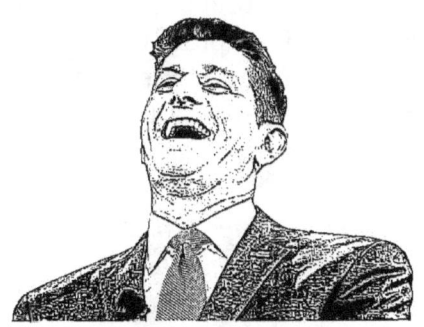

Paul Ryan
(Republican)
Speaker of the House

Many people think members of Congress (House of Representatives and the Senate) get the *__best__* health care coverage. They do!

Let's take a minute before moving forward to answer a few frequently asked questions about that coverage.

Question: If my Medicare benefits are about to be "reformed", I wonder what type of benefits my representative to Congress or the Senate receives?

Legitimate question. The good news is we have a recent report (June 17, 2015) from the Congressional Research Service on just this question. The report was prepared for Members and Committees of Congress. One thing we learn is that prior to 2014, Members had access to many of the same health benefits as other federal employees through the Federal Employee Health Benefits (FEHB) program. All that changed on January 1, 2014 with the implementation of new rules created under the Affordable Care Act (Obamacare if you must).

It certainly makes one wonder if these changes contribute to the fury and outright hatred by Republicans (and some Democrats) of the ACA. The Authors believe that this "forced" participation really gets under their skin. With repeal of the ACA, Congressional health insurance coverage would revert back to the FEHB program.

Since 2014, Congressional Members must enroll in a plan offered through a health exchange in order to receive a government contribution (between 72% and 75%) toward the cost of their premium. The exchange is called the DC Health Link and it has the following statement on the Health Link website: *"The outcome of the 2016 presidential election doesn't impact your ability to enroll in affordable quality health insurance for 2017. You may also be eligible for* **premium reductions**. *The DC Health Link has 20 private health insurance options to choose from for residents and their families from CareFirst (Blue Cross/Blue Shield) and Kaiser Permanente. For 2017 small businesses have 151 health plan options from Aetna, CareFirst, Kaiser, and United Healthcare."*

NOTE: Member and staff contributions to premiums are collected through payroll deductions and contributions are noted as "tax preferred".

There are an additional five benefits available to Members—all outside the ACA.

1. Federal Flexible Spending Account Program. This Program includes the Dependent Care Flexible Spending Account that reimburses eligible non-medical child day care and elder care expenses with a $5,000 limit. This account is paid through **pre-tax dollars** effectively lowering the final annual Federal taxable income.
2. Federal Employees Dental and Vision Insurance

Program. Members who enroll pay 100% of the premium through salary contributions with **pre-tax dollars**.

3. The third program is one that MOST health insurance plans **do not include**. This is the Federal Long Term Care Insurance Program with premiums deducted from the salary or annuity of the enrollee. The employee pays 100% of the premium. This Program has a **preferred tax status**. The Federal Long Term Care Insurance Program is designed to be a tax-qualified plan under the Internal Revenue Code.

4. Members of Congress are also eligible to receive services from the Office of the Attending Physician for an annual fee (2016 - $611). These services include routine exams, consultations and diagnostic tests. The present Attending Physician is a Rear Admiral (Navy) who graduated from Georgetown Medical School and has specialties in Internal Medicine and Hematology/Oncology.

5. Any Member of Congress is authorized to received medical and emergency dental care at military treatment facilities (inpatient or outpatient) located within the National Capital Region—whether they have served in the military or not.

Question: "What about Medicare for Members of Congress?"

Under the current Congressional health care coverage, Members of Congress may carry both Medicare and an individual Health Care Exchange policy.

What this means in plain English is that Congress gets to "double-dip" and *you don't*.

A History Of Medicare

So, let's have a Medicare history lesson. The best place to start is from the beginning. Listed below are nine key dates in the history of Medicare and the related laws. You can get your cup of coffee after you read this section. It's important. And it's short.

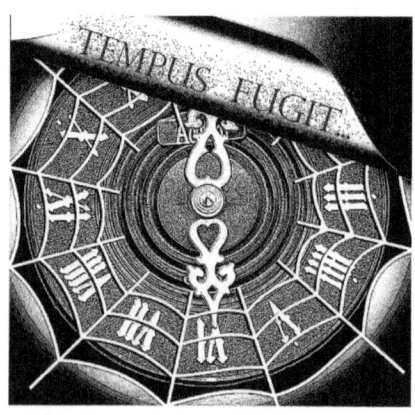

As far as we can tell, the idea of Universal Healthcare originated with Teddy Roosevelt via his Progressive Bull Moose Party in 1912. His vision included:
- A National Health Service
- Social Insurance for the elderly, the unemployed and the disabled
- Worker's Compensation for work-related injuries

...and yes, more. Then came those who followed...

Timeline

1945: It was President Truman (Democrat) who first sent a message to Congress, on November 19, 1945, calling for the creation of a national health insurance fund, **open to all Americans**. Truman fought throughout his presidential term to get the bill passed but he was unsuccessful.

1962: In the spring of 1962, President John F. Kennedy (Democrat) launched his effort to provide health care for the aged. His effort peaked in a nationally televised address from Madison Square Garden--it was a flop. The legislation foundered amid charges by the Republicans that it was an attempt to socialize medicine.

1965: On July 30, 1965 President Johnson (Democrat) signed the bill that would become Medicare known as "Original Medicare" covering Part A (hospital insurance) and Part B (medical insurance).

1972: President Nixon (Republican) signed the *Social Security Amendments of 1972* on October 30 of that year providing Medicare insurance to those who had been severely disabled for over two years, coverage to people with End Stage Renal Disease (ESRD), and raising the Medicare payroll tax.

1980: The Democratic-led Congress passed the

Omnibus Reconciliation Act that expanded home health services under Medicare and brought Medigap (Medicare supplemental insurance program) under federal oversight.

1997: The Medicare Part C (Managed Care) program was created by the *Balanced Budget Act of 1997* and signed into law by Congress on August 5. In order to reduce Medicare spending, the act reduced payments to health service providers such as hospitals, doctors, and nurse practitioners. It was originally known as Medicare+Choice (M+C), and was designed to provide coverage through private insurers beyond that under Medicare Parts A and B and at a lower cost to the Medicare beneficiary.

2003: President George W. Bush (Republican) signed the *Medicare Prescription Drug Improvement and Modernization Act* on December 8, 2003 and said, "With the Medicare Act of 2003, our government is finally bringing prescription drug coverage to the seniors of America. With this law, we're giving older Americans better choices and more control over their health care, so they can receive the modern medical care they deserve. With this law, we are providing more access to comprehensive exams, disease screenings, and other preventative care, so that seniors across this land can live better and healthier lives."

2010: On March 23, 2010, President Obama (Democrat) signed the *Patient Protection and Affordable Care Act (ACA) of 2010* that included a long list of reform provisions to contain Medicare costs while increasing revenue, improving and streamlining Medicare delivery systems, and increasing services within the program.

—Okay, now you can get your cup of coffee.

Funding of Medicare

How is Medicare paid?

This section is a bit "tricky", you might even get bored, but hang in there with us.

So... let's follow the money.

Medicare is paid for through two trust funds (a fund made up of several types of assets intended to provide benefits to an individual or organization). The two funds are The Hospital Insurance trust (HI) fund and the Supplemental Medical Insurance (SMI) trust fund. The HI trust fund finances Medicare Part A, and collects its revenue primarily through a payroll tax on all U.S. workers and employers.

The Social Security Act established the Medicare Board of Trustees to oversee the financial operations of the HI and SMI trust funds. The Board has six members. Four members serve by virtue of their positions in the Federal Government: the Secretary of the Treasury, who is the Managing Trustee; the Secretary of Labor; the

Secretary of Health and Human Services; and the Commissioner of Social Security. Two other members are public representatives whom the President appoints and the Senate confirms. These positions are currently vacant. The Administrator of the Centers for Medicare & Medicaid Services (CMS) serves as Secretary of the Board.

The SMI trust fund finances both voluntary Medicare programs – Part B (medical insurance) and Part D (drug insurance). Funding for this trust comes mostly from premiums paid by Medicare members and general revenues. Unlike the HI fund, there are no dedicated payroll taxes for the SMI. Instead, the fund's chief revenue sources are contributions from the general fund (receipts from other sources, such as individual income taxes, corporate taxes, and excise taxes), premiums from participants (there are separate premiums for Parts B and D), and a small amount of interest on trust fund balances and miscellaneous receipts.

Part C (managed care insurance) is paid for through funds from both the HI and SMI trust funds, and collects its revenues from a combination of general revenues, payroll taxes, beneficiary premiums, and out-of-pocket charges.

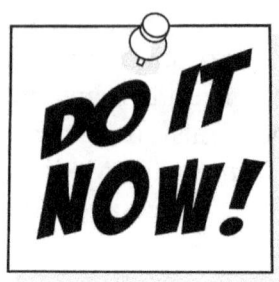

READ THESE FACTS

As of February 2014, the assessed Medicare tax rate:

Employer pays	1.45%
Employee pays	1.45%

Yes, higher income folks do pay a little more in taxes, 0.9% in fact. They can afford it. These employees are earning at least $200,000 individually or a combined married income of $250,000 or more. However, there is NO matching employer tax rate. .

It is a FACT that each of us pays into the HI program directly through taxes collected from the first day we go to work. Yes, **YOU** pay for Medicare…you have been paying for years! You ARE entitled to receive Medicare because you have been paying for Medicare you entire working life.

It is also a FACT that each of us pays for Medicare Parts B and D through our individual income taxes and our premiums. You ARE entitled to receive Medicare medical and drug benefits because you have been paying individual taxes to support these two programs and when you become eligible you will continue to support the program through premium payments and other out-of-pocket costs such as deductibles.

The Authors feel that the following chart, courtesy of the *Kaiser Family Foundation* article best illustrates what we're trying to say. Thank you Kaiser.

HOW IS MEDICARE FINANCED?

Medicare is funded primarily from three sources: general revenues (41%), payroll taxes (38%), and beneficiary premiums (13%) **(Figure 6)**.

Figure 6

Sources of Medicare Revenue, 2014

41%	1%		
	87%	73%	74%
38%			
		25%	15%
13%	1%		11%
1%	1%		
2%	7%	1%	
1%	3%	1%	1%
TOTAL	**Part A**	**Part B**	**Part D**
$599.3 billion	$261.2 billion	$259.8 billion	$78.2 billion

- General revenue
- Payroll taxes
- Premiums
- Transfers from states
- Taxation of Social Security benefits
- Interest
- Other

NOTE Data are for the calendar year.
SOURCE: 2015 Annual Report of the Boards of Trustees of the Federal Hospital Insurance and Federal Supplementary Medical Insurance Trust Funds.

THE HENRY J
KAISER
FAMILY
FOUNDATION

Agencies In Charge Of Medicare

There are three key government agencies that oversee Medicare benefits and enrollment. We're including a list and brief description because we think it's important for you to know. It's part of the picture.

Social Security is an independent federal agency with a seven member bipartisan advisory board. The administration of the Medicare program is a responsibility of the Centers for Medicare and Medicaid Services, but SSA offices are used for determining initial eligibility, some processing of premium payments, and for limited public contact information. They also administer a financial needs-based program which supplements Medicare Part D (drug insurance) program enrollees. Its central office is located in Baltimore, Maryland.

Department of Health and Human Services (DHHS) is headed by a Secretary who is part of the President's Cabinet. The Department oversees eleven agencies including the Food and Drug Administration (FDA), Center for Disease Control (CDC), National Institutes of Health (NIH), Administration for Children and Families (ACF) and Centers for Medicare & Medicaid Services (CMS).

Centers for Medicare and Medicaid Services (CMS) is charged primarily with implementing policies and managing the day-to-day Medicare program including processing hospital and medical claims. CMS is a Federal agency within the Department of Health and Human Services and has over 6,000 employees— primarily located in its Maryland headquarters. That said, CMS has 10 regional offices – Boston, New York City, Philadelphia, Atlanta, Chicago, Dallas, Kansas City, Denver, San Francisco and Seattle.

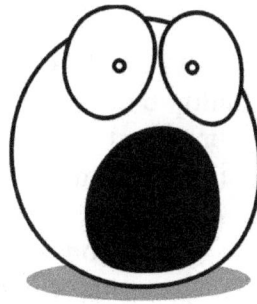

The two key areas responsible for implementing Medicare related policies are DHHS and CMS. The Secretary of DHHS and the Administrator of CMS are appointed by the President and confirmed by the Senate. Let's take a look at who Trump has chosen for these two offices...

DHHS Secretary – Tom Price

Representative Price assumed office in January 2005 from Georgia's 6th district (Atlanta). Price proudly participates in the Association of American Physicians and Surgeons (2014 membership was roughly 5,000 members) a politically conservative association organized to "fight socialized medicine and to fight the government takeover of medicine". The AAPS is often in conflict with the better known American Medical Association (AMA) (2013 membership roughly 228,000 members) due to the AAPS's conservative agenda. For example the AMA supported the passage of Obamacare (if I must).

As one would expect, Mr. Price voted for repeal of the ACA (if **you** insist, Obamacare) on multiple occasions, opposes abortion and supported the proposed Protect Life Act (2011), and voted against a bill that prohibited job discrimination based on sexual orientation. He received a "0" rating from Planned Parenthood and NARAL Pro-Choice America; a 0% approval rating from the Brady Campaign to Prevent Gun Violence; and a 0% rating by the Human Rights Campaign.

He sponsored the *Empowering Patients First Act* (EPFA) in Congress that was intended to be the Republican alternative to the Affordable Care Act while serving with Mike Pence on the regressive Republican Study Committee.

Speaking of Pence…

CMS Administrator selection – Seema Verma

Ms. Verma has built a health policy consulting company - Seema Verma Consultants (SVC) and consults with conservative Republican Governors to "reform" their state Medicaid programs. In the opinion of the Authors, "reform" being used as a code word for decreasing benefits and increasing the cost of Medicaid for those least likely to be able to afford it. We expect to see the same type of "reforms" at the national level. Watch for code words such as modernization, reform, empowering, health care savings, better choices, increased access, etc.

The work she has done in Kentucky requires all Medicaid recipients to work—she calls it the "skin in the game" clause. This is similar to the requirement in Indiana that recipients pay premiums and have their access restricted if they fail to pay on time. Oh yes, the hospitals and doctors in Indiana are delighted with these changes because they saw Medicaid reimbursements go up 20% and 25% respectively. So, in plain English, hospitals got a 20% raise and doctors got a 25% raise. You get the bill.

An article in *The Indianapolis Star* raises concerns over a potential conflict of interest from Verma's roles as *both* a health care consultant for Indiana and an employee of a Hewlett-Packard division that is among Indiana's largest Medicaid vendors. By 2014 SVC Inc. (Verma's company) had been awarded over $3.5 million in Indiana state contracts. During that same time period, Verma was employed with Hewlett-Packard, earning over $1 million during the same period in which the company had secured $500 million in state contracts.

Do you think these two people have the best interests of Medicare and it's beneficiaries (that would be you) as their primary consideration?

Let's Talk

Medicare's "Alphabet Soup"

Medicare has four program "parts," offering three types of health coverage:
1. Part A   Hospital
2. Part B   Medical
3. Part C   HMO and PPO
4. Part D   Drugs

Almost all Americans are automatically enrolled in Part A *at no additional cost* once they turn 65 years old. Medicare Parts B, C, and D are *voluntary* and require those who enroll to pay premiums in order to receive coverage.

Medicare Part A – the hospital program covers hospital care, skilled nursing facility care, nursing home care (non-custodial), hospice, and home health services

Medicare Part B – the outpatient program covers (1) medically necessary services OR supplies needed to diagnose or treat a medical condition and that meet accepted standards of medical practice and (2) health care services to prevent illness (flu) OR detect illness at an early stage. Some examples of Part B services include: primary care and specialty doctor office visits, medical equipment, outpatient services at the hospital, laboratory testing, mental health services, and ambulance.

Medicare Part C – the part of the Medicare program that allows *private* health insurance companies to provide Medicare benefits through health plans, such as HMOs (Health Maintenance Organization) and PPOs (Preferred Provider Organization). The largest *private health insurance plans* offering HMOs and PPOs in 2016 are United Healthcare, Humana, Blue Cross/Blue Shield and Kaiser Permanente.

Medicare Part D – the program designed to subsidize the costs of prescription drugs and prescription drug insurance premiums for Medicare beneficiaries.

Future pamphlets will cover in detail each type of Medicare program as well as Medicare supplemental insurance program options.

A Few "Big Picture" Facts

At this point, we thought it would be helpful to insert a few facts about Medicare, the number enrolled, and the number enrolled by "type" of enrollment – age and disability. Below are some "hard" statistics from 2013 and 2016:

Fact #1: in 2013 Medicare enrollees = 52,506,598 or approximately 17.5% of the total US population.

Fact #2: in 2013 84% of Medicare enrollees were "aged" and 16% were "disabled".

Fact #3: 69% of Americans were enrolled in traditional Medicare and 31% were enrolled in Medicare Part C plans in 2016.

Fact #4: the States with the highest percentage of Medicare enrollments due to disability are in the Southern U.S. (see 2016 chart below).

State	Medicare Enrollment	% Aged	% Disabled
Louisiana	752,435	79%	21%
Arkansas	573,498	77%	23%
Mississippi	537,250	76%	24%
Alabama	922,695	76%	24%
Tennessee	1,170,888	79%	21%
Kentucky	827,163	75%	25%
W. Virginia	404,943	77%	23%

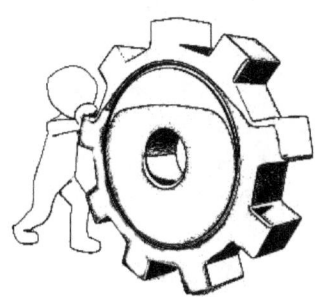

Who Gets Medicare?

Situation #1: If you are 65 or older and you are a citizen or a permanent resident of the United States you are eligible for Medicare Part A (hospital insurance) at *no cost* when:

- You receive OR are eligible to receive Social Security benefits;
- You receive OR are eligible to receive Railroad Retirement benefits;
- Your spouse (living or deceased including divorced spouses) receives OR is eligible to receive Social Security or Railroad Retirement benefits;
- You OR your spouse worked long enough in a government job and you paid Medicare taxes.

If you do not meet these requirements, you may be able to purchase Medicare Part A by paying a monthly premium. Don't forget—you have to be 65! As we've mentioned, most people don't pay a monthly premium for Part A (sometimes called "premium-free Part A"). If you buy Part A, you'll pay up to $413 each month. The premium is based on how many quarters you worked in your life. If you paid Medicare taxes for less than 30 quarters (7.5 years) , the standard Part A premium is $413. If you paid Medicare taxes for 30-39 quarters (up to 9.75 years), the standard Part A premium is $227.

Situation #2: Before you are 65 or older, you are eligible for Medicare Part A (hospital insurance) at *no cost* when:

- You have been entitled to Social Security disability for 24 months;
- You receive a disability pension from the Railroad Retirement Board;
- You receive Social Security disability benefits because you have Lou Gehrig's Disease;
- You worked long enough in a government job where you paid Medicare taxes and you have been entitled to Social Security disability benefits;
- You are the child or widow(er) (50 or older) including a divorced widow(er), of someone who has worked long enough in a government job where you have paid Medicare taxes and you are entitled to Social Security disability benefits;
- You have permanent kidney failure and you receive maintenance dialysis or have had a kidney transplant.

If you automatically quality for Medicare Part A (hospital insurance) at *no cost*, you qualify for Medicare Part B (medical insurance).   There is a monthly premium. If you are not eligible for Part A at *no cost* you can buy Part B—without having to buy Part A. In simple layman's terms, you pay a premium and get Part B (medical insurance):

1. If you are 65;
2. If you are a U.S. citizen;
3. If you are a lawfully admitted non-citizen who

has lived in the U.S. for at least 5 years.

We know this is complicated—hang in there!

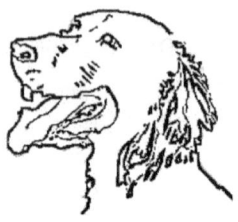

This might be a good time to insert a chart...here is one showing premium increases since the inception of Medicare.

MEDICARE PART B
MONTHLY PREMIUM HISTORY
(By Decade)

Date	Enrollee Pays (Aged & Disabled)	Government Pays – Aged	Government Pays – Disabled*
1966	$3.00	$3.00	$0
1970	$5.30	$5.30	$0
1980	$9.60	$23.00	$41.40
1990	$28.60	$85.80	$59.60
2000	$45.50	$138.30	$196.70
2010	$110.50	$331.50	$430.30

*Medicare for the disabled begins in 1972. The government pays $22.70 beginning in 1973.

So What's Up With The Premium Part B for 2017?

The standard Part B premium amount in 2017 should be $134 (or higher depending on your income). *__Most__* people who get Social Security benefits pay less than this amount as the Part B premium increased *__more than__* the cost-of-living increase for 2017 Social Security benefits. If you pay your Part B premium through your monthly Social Security benefit, the cost will be (on average) $109.

So, in plain English what this means is the true cost of the Part B premium for 2017 should be $134. However because the cost-of-living increase for Social Security is so low the true $25 increase could not be passed on to the average person receiving Social Security.

That $25 still has to come from somewhere. The Authors have no access to the information as to where that money will come from, whether it's from general taxes or some other source. Another question we cannot answer is, "What caused health care costs to create a whopping $25 premium increase from 2016 to 2017?" If we don't know, what makes us think it won't happen again this year...and the next?

Putting Some "Meat on the Bones" of Medicare

If you already receive Social Security benefits (or Railroad Retirement checks), Social Security will send you Medicare enrollment information a few months before you become eligible (your birth month). Even if your birthday is the last day of the month (January 31, for example) your effective date with Medicare is the first day of the month (in this case, January 1).

This information will include the "red, white and blue" Medicare card showing whether you have Part A (hospital), Part B (medical) or both. Laminate it. Keep it close. Give a copy to a trustworthy family member. This is your passport for all you basic health care benefits.

Because you pay a premium for Part B (medical coverage) you can choose to turn this insurance coverage down. (Instructions on how to turn it down are on the back of the Red White and Blue card you receive.)

1. Carry your card with you when you're away from home.
2. Let your hospital or doctor see your card when you need hospital, medical, or health services under **Medicare**.
3. Your card is good wherever you live in the United States.

WARNING: Issued only for use of the named beneficiary. Intentional misuse of this card is unlawful and may be punishable by fines, imprisonment, and other penalties. If found, drop in nearest U.S. Mail Box.

CMS

Centers for Medicare &
Medicaid Services
Baltimore, MD 21244-1850
Form CMS-40 (04/2013)

Questions about Medicare:
- visit Medicare.gov
- call 1-800-MEDICARE
  (1-800-633-4227);
  (TTY: 1-877-486-2048)

I DO NOT WANT MEDICAL INSURANCE ☐ Check Here

	Written Signature (or Legal Representative)
SIGN HERE	
	Signature by Mark (✖) Must Be Witnessed
Signature of Witness	
Address of Witness	

If you do NOT want Part B (Medical Insurance):

1. Check the box above (top right), sign your name, and return the entire form in the enclosed envelope. Do NOT tear off the Medicare card. You must return the form BEFORE the Part B effective date shown on the card.

2. You still have Part A even though you do not want Part B. We will send you a new card showing that you have Part A only. If you need Medicare services before your new card arrives, you can tell the provider that you have Medicare or show the letter you got from Social Security telling you about your new Medicare coverage.

Important! In most cases, if you don't sign up for Medicare Part B (Medical Insurance) when you're first eligible, you'll have to pay a late enrollment penalty for as long as you have Part B. Also, you may have to wait until the Medicare General Enrollment Period (from January 1 to March 31) to enroll in Part B and coverage will start July 1 of that year.

To learn more about when you can enroll and the penalty, visit Medicare.gov, see your Medicare & You handbook, or call 1-800-MEDICARE (1-800-633-4227). TTY users should call: 1-877-486-2048.

Part B (Medical Insurance)

When first eligible for Medicare Part A (hospital insurance) each individual has a 7-month period to sign up for Part B (medical insurance).

This is called the Initial Enrollment Period (IEP). If you are eligible for Medicare because of a medical disability, the IEP depends on the date your disability begins. This pamphlet focuses primarily on the enrollment for those 65 and over.

If you enroll	Part B Coverage Begins
1 to 3 months before your 65th birth month	Your birth month
Your birth month	1 month after your birth month
1 month after your birth month	2 months after the birth month
2 to 3 months after your birth month	3 months after birth month

Examples really helps…Enrollee turns 65 in month of March (birth month):

Enroll	Part B Coverage Begins
December (3 months before), January (2 months before) or February (1 month before)	March 1
March – birth month	April 1
April – 1 month after birth month	May 1
May or June – 2 to 3 months after birth month	June 1

We know…we know…tedious but important— particularly this next bit.

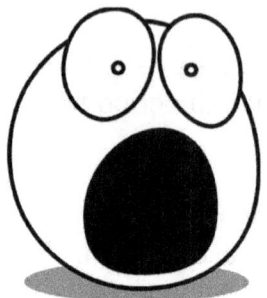

Yes indeed...there is a Part A Late Enrollment Penalty!

Don't forget: If you are not eligible for a _**no cost**_ Part A (hospital insurance) and you do not buy Part A when you are first eligible, you may pay a Late Enrollment Penalty—as much as 10%. You will pay the higher premium for 2 times the number of years you could have been enrolled in Part A but you did not sign up!

So...for example...you could have enrolled in Part A but did not until 2 years later. You would pay the higher premium for a total of 4 years unless you have a Special Enrollment Period (SEP).

_If_ you do not enroll in Part B (medical insurance) when you are first eligible, you may have to pay a Late Enrollment Penalty (LEP) unless you qualify for a Special Election Period (SEP). If you do not have a SEP, the late enrollment penalty _**never goes away**_ (you pay it every month) for as long as you have Part B medical insurance. Details about SEP's are available at www.Medicare.gov.

Want An Example Of A Part B Late Enrollment Penalty?

You have an Initial Enrollment Period (IEP) that ended on September 30, 2015. You waited to sign up for Part B until the General Enrollment Period (GEP). The GEP lasts from January 1 to March 31 every year. You chose to enroll in February, 2017 (one full year and five months late). Your monthly premium penalty is 10% for *each* 12-month period that you could have had Part B but didn't sign up for it.

In dollars…the 2017 base premium is $109 (for most people). Add the penalty of one 10% twelve month period (approximately $10.90) to reach your premium amount of $119.90. ***This penalty never goes away.*** You will have to pay the 10% penalty as long as you have Part B. The 10% penalty is always based on the current year premium.

JUST SO WE ARE CRYSTAL CLEAR… If you weren't automatically enrolled in Medicare, you missed your IEP, and you do not have an SEP, you can still apply for Medicare Part A (hospital insurance) and/or Medicare Part B (medical insurance) during the General Enrollment Period (GEP), which runs from January 1 to March 31 each year. If you enroll in Medicare during the General Enrollment Period, your coverage begins on July 1.

The rules for these three types of enrollment periods are not the same:

- IEP - Seven month period-three months before the birth month, the birth month and three months after the birth month, specific to each individual.
- OEP (Open Enrollment Period) – October 15 through December 7, every year.
- GEP – January 1 to March 31, every year .

General Enrollment Period

Those eligible for Medicare Part A (hospital insurance) and Medicare Part B (medical insurance) can sign up during the General Enrollment Period (GEP). This period occurs every year between January 1 and March 31 when one of these circumstances apply:

- You did not sign up when first eligible;
- You do not have a Special Enrollment Period (SEP);
- You must pay premiums for Part A and/or Part B.

Coverage is effective on July 1.

Special Enrollment Period

If you are covered under a group health plan based on current employment, there is a SEP to sign up for Part A and/or Part B as long as the following applies: (1) you or your spouse (or a family member if you are disabled) is working and (2) you are covered by a group health plan through an employer or union.

You will be given an 8-month SEP to sign up for Part A and/or Part B that begins on one of the following: (1) the month after employment ends OR (2) the month after group health plan insurance based on current employment ends.

Question: Why is enrollment so complicated? This is a legitimate question and one many people ask. Let's try to give a couple of pretty clear answers.

Answer: First, there are two agencies involved in Medicare – Social Security and the Centers for Medicare and Medicaid Services (better known in its abbreviated form—CMS). These agencies share information but not databases resulting in delays in sharing information. Social Security houses information on key components of Medicare enrollment: (1) eligibility due to age, (2) social security numbers, and (3) data on contributions to Medicare through taxes.

Gotta have this information if you are going to enroll!

On the other hand, CMS runs the day-to-day operations of Medicare from enrollment to paying claims. You cannot be enrolled without a social security number and claims cannot be paid for your healthcare unless you can be linked to a member number. Pretty simple.

Yes, you get to carry around that red-white and blue card plus your insurance card—and perhaps a separate Part D prescription card depending on the choices you have made.

Believe me it gets even more complicated when you add in the Part C (managed care insurance) and Part D (drug insurance) enrollment process!

Second, let's use an example to help clarify. My birthday is in March. I have an "initial enrollment period" for the 3 months prior to my birth month, my birth month, and 3 months after my birth month—December through June. That's a long time. But…you know people…they wait, they procrastinate, they lose their forms, and they need help. So this time frame was established to *make it easier* for newly eligible Medicare people to first enroll. It is definitely not a conspiracy—though it may sometimes feel like one.

Another question: Why are there penalties for not enrolling?

Answer: Honestly, I don't know the workings of the minds of bureaucrats but let me take a couple of guesses. First, the more people enrolled in an insurance program the larger the pool of people to spread costs among—that is what insurance is all about—the numbers...and the costs of course. If you are a healthy 65 year old, not going to the doctor and not using prescription medicine, Medicare is going to want your healthy body to add to its much older and more costly users. By charging a late enrollment penalty Medicare will push more people to enroll and spread the costs around.

Final Words

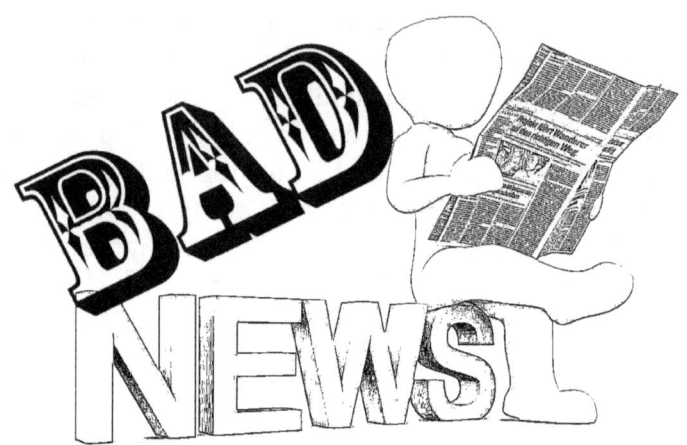

<u>Reality Can Be Brutal</u>

The future of Medicare (maybe *your* Medicare) has never been under the level of threat that it faces today. "Why? You might ask." The pot of gold set aside to pay Medicare benefits is so big that it is too tempting to health care corporations to leave alone. And, honestly… the ability to fund the program is becoming more challenging without asking for increased taxes on the wealthy and more cost sharing on the part of all enrollees.

We all know why it is becoming more difficult to fund the program but let's make a list anyway:

1. The population is *aging*;
2. The number of disabled applying and receiving Medicare coverage is *growing*;
3. The aging population is *living longer*;
4. Heath care *costs are increasing*;
5. As average income *stalls or drops* the amount collected in the "Medicare tax" to fund the Hospital Insurance (HI) trust goes down.

Some numbers from the National Health Expenditures (NHE) Fact Sheet provides a bit of perspective:

- Medicare spending grew by 4.5% in 2012 to $646.2 billion dollars.
- Health care spending on a per person basis for those 65 and older was $18,988 or *5 times higher* than spending per child ($3,552) and *3 times higher* than spending for working-aged persons ($6,632).
- The elderly are the smallest population group (approximately 14% of the total U.S. population) but accounted for approximately 34% of all health spending in 2012.

Let's get real...something about this picture is going to have to change. Or maybe even many "somethings". Yet with all its flaws and concerns about Medicare's "financial health" it works for over 50 million people and it could be changed to meet the needs of all Americans.

Yes, we can do it!

At the beginning of the pamphlet we promised to meet two goals:

First Goal – Educate the Reader

We believe we met the goal! Let's put the highlights here:

- We explained how Medicare gets is money and how *you* contribute to that pool of dollars – remember that 1.45% tax on your income (and the matching amount from the employer not visible on your pay stub)? Yeah that one. So in 2014 87% of *all* Medicare Part A (hospital insurance) revenue dollars were obtained from payroll taxes.

- We talked about how Social Security and the Centers for Medicare and Medicaid Services (CMS) work closely together to identify those eligible for enrollment. I hope our Readers recall the brief explanation of the four Medicare Programs—"alphabet soup".

- Because each of those four programs (hospital insurance, medical insurance, managed care insurance and drug insurance) are so complicated we will be devoting 3 more pamphlets explaining how they work, how they are funded and proposed changes to each program.

- Because the situation is changing so quickly, the facts presented in each pamphlet will be those that are relevant on the date the pamphlet goes to press.

- Finally, we gave the Reader a lengthy discussion on how enrollment in Medicare works—for those 65 and older. You have to love those "initials": GEP, IEP, SEP, LEP, etc. Our apologies to the disabled but we wanted to get this pamphlet in the hands of our Readers and did not have time to talk about Medicare disability enrollment. (Another day. Another pamphlet).

Second Goal – Call to Action (CTA)

Medicare is under fire right this minute. On a daily basis our Facebook inboxes are filled with articles about various "reform" proposals using lots of misleading language meant to frighten current Medicare enrollees or to deflect from the truth.

- *Whenever* anyone talks about "reform" they

really mean decreasing funding.

- *Whenever* anyone talks about increasing access they really mean limiting access through selected provider networks (herding you into pens like sheep).
- *Whenever* anyone talks about "premium support" they really mean setting a premium maximum wherein all costs above that support number are on the shoulders of the Medicare enrollee.
- *Whenever* anyone uses the word "voucher" it makes me think about my "Harry's Roadhouse" coupon that covers a maximum dinner-for-two of $40 while everything above that it out-of-my-pocket.

As we emphasized in the Introduction, we all need to DO SOMETHING (or several somethings) to hold on to the current program—and possibly extend it to all Americans.   After all, over 55 million people are currently enrolled and are pretty happy with their insurance coverage. Let's suggest some "easy" stuff and then some "harder" stuff.

The Easy Stuff:

CTA#1: Ok…this is simple…get out your latest pay stub. That 1.45% tax you pay for Medicare has its own line and generally appears after Federal and State taxes and is simply called "Medicare Tax". Now you have proven to yourself that you are indeed contributing to the cost of Medicare. If you are not currently working, ask one of your kids to look at their pay stub. Even better...do it with them. They need to learn about this too.

CTA#2: Medicare is not free! We are adding this link http://bit.ly/MedicareCosts2017 where you can see the additional Part A (hospital insurance) and Part B (medical insurance) costs for 2017. What? I thought Medicare Part A was at *no cost*? True. There is no added premium but there is that pesky $1316 deductible per year for each benefit period! (You read that right – you're responsible for that amount IN ADDITION to your monthly premiums).

The Harder Stuff:

CTA#3: Want to get political? Write (letter or postcard), e-mail or call the new Secretary of Health and Human Services (Tom Price) and tell him *not to* support privatization of health care. If you really want to do something, tell Trump the same thing.

We have attached a draft letter found in the EXTRAS section of this pamphlet. If you have a desire to do more you can send the same letter to your Senators and the Congressperson from your district.

Contact the Department of Health and Human Services:
200 Independence Avenue, S.W.
Washington, D.C. 20201
Toll Free Call Center: 1-877-696-6775
http://bit.ly/HHSContact

Contact the White House:
Comments: 202-456-1111
Switchboard: 202-456-1414
Address: 1600 Pennsylvania Ave NW, Washington, DC 20500

CTA#4: Check out the chart below to see how Part B (medical insurance) premiums have increased over the 5 decades since the beginning of Medicare in 1966. You may recall there is not currently an additional Part A (hospital insurance) premium as the Medicare tax you pay plus general revenue funds have been adequate to cover these costs. The repeal of the ACA (oh, please! Obamacare) would significantly speed up the projected insolvency of the Hospital Insurance trust fund— remember Part A benefits are paid from this fund. For those of you who do not know what "insolvency" means, it is not having enough money in your checking account to cover your water company bill.

Time Period	Enrollee Premium Dollar Amount Increase	Enrollee Premium Percentage Increase
1966-1970	$2.30	56%
1971-1980	$4.30	55%
1981-1990	$19.00	33%
1991-2000	$16.90	63%
2000-2010	$60.50	41%

Final Words

Our final CTA, write, e-mail or call your representatives http://www.house.gov/representatives/find/ and tell them you want them to keep the additional Medicare tax on higher income earners. We drafted another letter to make this task as easy as possible. (It's at the end with the EXTRAS).

Let's Get Real

The ACA, and its Medicare funding and quality reforms, is pretty much going to go away and a lot sooner than most of us could have believed. We need to say "goodbye" and mourn its death. Inserted here is a link to a well-written Kaiser Foundation article describing the repeal (and or defunding) impact on the Medicare program. Certainly something to chew on. http://kaiserf.am/2kOo2NO

When the ACA is fully repealed (or just flat out defunded) and replaced (or *not replaced* by a back-to-the-future vision), making Medicare private is next on the agenda. Remember that the new Secretary of Health and Human Services, Tom Price, is a *YUGE* fan of the Medicare voucher system. Price will now be in a position to push Trump to drop his pledge:

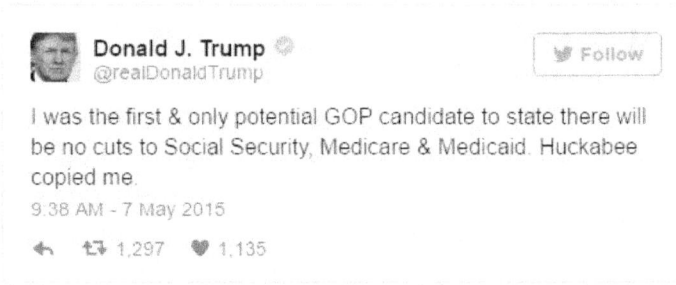

Donald J. Trump
@realDonaldTrump

🔲 Follow

I was the first & only potential GOP candidate to state there will be no cuts to Social Security, Medicare & Medicaid. Huckabee copied me.

9:38 AM - 7 May 2015

↩ ♺ 1,297 ♥ 1,135

The Authors believe it is just wrong-headed to make any changes to Medicare at this time—except to offer it to every American.

Let's be honest…Politicians in charge of preserving and ensuring Medicare's continuation are bought and paid for by corporations and, as we learned early in the pamphlet, have pretty darn good health insurance to boot. They might look like Goliath, they might yell like Goliath, they might try to make you afraid like Goliath but by getting educated and taking action you CAN have a voice.

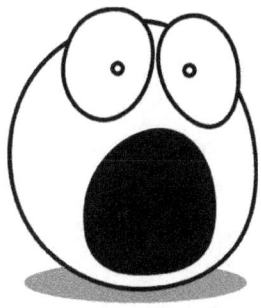

COMING SOON!

Medicare is complicated as we've said before. This is why we've chosen bite size doses of information in the form of pamphlets.

Next up is a pamphlet that talks only about Medicare Part A (Hospital Insurance) and Medicare Part B (Medical Insurance) in great detail.

Following that will be a pamphlet on Medicare Part C (Managed Care Insurance), and then another pamphlet devoted entirely to Medicare Part D (Drug insurance). Yes, it's required. Yes, you pay a premium for it.

We will continue to tackle other Medicare subjects beyond these four pamphlets and will be initiating a blog where you can ask questions and get current information. You can expect a new pamphlet approximately every six weeks.

EXTRAS
Contact Your Senator

If you have not emailed your Senator before - it's easy if you go step by step.

Step 1: **GO** to this link
https://www.senate.gov/senators/contact/

Step 2: click on Senator's phone list (the third box down on the right)

Step 3. You will find Senators alphabetically by last name, a column with their party affiliation and state and a column with their phone number.

 Happy calling!

Contact Your Representative

Step 1: **GO** to this link
 http://www.house.gov/representatives/find/

Step 2: Enter your 5 digit zip code and click the red button: Find Your Rep By Zip

Step 3: Find your Representative's Washington DC phone number at the bottom of the page.

 Happy calling!

Letter to Secretary of Health and Human Services

Tom Price
Secretary of Health and Human Services
Department of Health and Human Services
200 Independence Avenue, S.W.
Washington, D.C. 20201

Dear Mr. Secretary:

Today Medicare works for over 55 million people. Let's not change that!

As a concerned citizen, I am urging you ***not to*** support the privatization of Medicare.

Respectfully,

Letter to President

Donald Trump, President
1600 Pennsylvania Ave NW
Washington, DC 20500

Dear Mr. Trump:

Today Medicare works for over 55 million people. Let's not change that! In fact, let's consider expanding Medicare to every American citizen.

We urge you to keep your campaign promise. On May 7, 2015 you tweeted, "I was the first and only potential GOP candidate to state there will be no cuts to Social Security, Medicare and Medicaid. Huckabee copied me."

Many people voted for you because of this one promise. Don't cave to pressure. A healthy America depends on you.

Sincerely,

Letter to Senator or Representative

Office of Senator (Name)
United States Senate
Washington, D.C. 20510

And

Office of Representative (Name)
U.S. House of Representatives
Washington, DC 20515

Dear (Name):

I am urging you _**to keep**_ the additional Medicare Tax (.9%) included in the Affordable Care Act. This is the tax on higher income earners. This tax will enable the Hospital Insurance Trust Fund to remain solvent until at least 2028.

Respectfully,